BAHASA UPDATE FOR DOCTORS
a Compilation of Articles from Berita MMA

EDARIAH ABU BAKAR

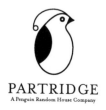

PARTRIDGE
A Penguin Random House Company

To order additional copies of this book, contact
Toll Free 800 101 2657 (Singapore)
Toll Free 1 800 81 7340 (Malaysia)
orders.singapore@partridgepublishing.com

www.partridgepublishing.com/singapore

INTRODUCING 'BAHASA UPDATE'

Malaysia's policy of unifying the various races through a common language, namely Bahasa Malaysia, has been implemented for several decades now with a good measure of success. But its twin goal of making B Malaysia a language of knowledge, the sciences and the professions, still lies far away beyond the horizons, though not quite unreachable.

The Bahasa Update

While most people in the medical profession (and recently prominent figures in politics) recognize the importance of English for our continuing education, we cannot run away from our commitment to mastering B Malaysia if we claim to be loyal citizens of this country. Most of us are humble enough to admit there is plenty of room for improvement in our daily and official communication. This is a crucial step in the right direction. The next is to do something about it. For this reason, Berita MMA will try to keep members up-to-date with Bahasa terminology, especially those relevant to the field and practice of medicine, through a regular 'Bahasa Update' column. To make it more meaningful and comprehensible, I will broach the subject from the angle of concepts and ideas, rather than merely provide an endless listing of what might appear to be 'misspelt English terms'. We won't go too heavy (we'll take the 'light-headed' approach). A pretest which you can try out will be offered on and off (to add some excitement and a dash of nostalgia to the good old exam blues of yesteryears) and a post-mortem feedback will be given . . . . in English, of course! (What better way to learn B Malaysia than through English? . . . and vice versa).

For starters . . .

Why not have a bash at the following jargon? . . . and see if you need to follow-up this Bahasa column regularly! All you have to do is to provide the technical and layman terms in Bahasa Malaysia for the English terms listed below, and check out your answers as provided. Give yourself one mark for each correct answer. (No need to minus marks for wrong ones!)

English Terms	Technical BM	Lay BM
ejaculation		
leg		
foot		
hookworm		
drug		
palpitations		
edema		
palate		
jaundice		
anxiety		

Answers *(Correct at the time of writing!)*

English Terms	Technical BM	Lay BM
ejaculation	*ejakulasi*	*pancutan*
leg	*tungkai*	*kaki*
foot	*kaki*	ditto
hookworm	*cacing kait*	ditto
drug	*dadah*	*ubat*
palpitations	*debaran*	ditto

edema	*edema*	sembab
palate	*lelangit*	ditto
jaundice	*jaundis*	*sakit kuning*
anxiety	*keresahan*	*resah/gelisah*

Verdict on Performance

* If you score 0-9, you should not miss out any issue of Berita MMA and gobble up this column. (I know you're a busy GP on the way up, but policy is policy).
* If you score 10-16, ... not bad, very promising. This column will pep you up!!
* If you score 17-20, **you** should be writing this column, not me!!! (Heck, I'm not even an MMA member).

Hopefully . . .

we will all benefit from this column. Yes . . . we . . . for I am a far cry from the versatile Adibah Amin. And the only way for me to maximize the benefit for you is to be given feedback on the running of the column, so it will be more palatable, and more importantly, effective to most, if not all, of us! Till we meet again next month, adios!!!

*   *   *

SCIENTIFIC VERSUS LAY

The Need for Scientific Medical Bahasa Malaysia

The last Update illustrated the existence of **scientific** or **technical** medical language as opposed to the language of the **lay** people. However, the need for scientific B Malaysia terminologies is not obvious to linguistic purists. They wonder why we do not use pure Malay words for all medical terms . . . . why not

5

pembedahan apendiks rather than ***apendektomi* (appendectomy)?** The superiority of the latter should be crystal clear to everyone. For one thing, *pembedahan apendiks* is not even a terminology, it is a definition!

Postmortem of the First Update

Let's recap the previous list:

Pancutan is not used as a scientific term for **ejaculation *(ejakulasi)*** because it literally means fountain. If we think about how a fountain works (24 hours a day by the gallons), it will immediately become obvious to us why *pancutan* is not acceptable as no man (not even Superman) can live up to this extraphysiological feat . . . of *pancut*-ing! (Anyone claiming to be capable, please report immediately to the Sperm Bank for the 70 million project!) But then language is such a dynamic thing . . . what's frowned upon today will become the high fashion of tomorrow. So who knows . . . future ejaculations might become *pancutan*s!

Tungkai **(leg)** had to be resuscitated from near-death (due to non-use) when anatomists had to keep on qualifying . . . *kaki* **(foot)** or *kaki* **(leg).** This state-of-affairs won't do at all, as it is not good for our linguistic image, not to mention the confusion plus-plus suffered by our poor medical students!

Hookworm is *cacing kait*, whether you're talking to a bunch of parasitologists or your *Mak Cik* from Ulu Kancong. Unfortunately, the Mistry-of-Health people had also baptized the **pinworm** as *cacing kait* when it should be *cacing kerawit*. (We can't very well blame the two worms for this mix-up, can we?) But not to worry . . . this will be sorted out once the *Kamus Perubatan* hits all three Campuses (and not forgetting, the Ministry of Health!).

You should never ask a mother whether her son *"ada makan/ambil dadah?"* when you're taking the **drug** history, for mother (and son) will never set foot in your clinic again! You should enquire instead whether the son *"ada makan ubat? . . .".* Legally, *dadah* is considered as **narcotic** drugs (not just 'drugs') by the authorities, no matter how pharmacologists tried to make them see that even good old panadol is a drug, and therefore a *dadah* . . . but this they refuse to accept as they have narrowed the concept of drugs to narcotics. Now *dadah* is further qualified by the word *najis* which laypeople (at least the not-too-religious ones) use for **feces**.

Palate cannot undergo the overprescribed treatment of mere spellchange to *palat*, as this would not be polite! So it is *lelangit* for both technical and lay usage.

Sakit kuning cannot be used for **jaundice** in scientific communication because it might be mistaken for yellow fever. However, to prevent the sudden onset of iatrogenic zombie facies in your patients, this (*sakit kuning*) is what you should use instead of insisting on finding out whether "*Encik ada **jaundis**?*"

For Effective Communication . . . .

It is obvious from the above discussion that we have to be well-versed in both the technical and lay terms. Communication within the scientific community via seminars, case presentations, educational or research publications, etc warrants the use of a scientific language, be it B Malaysia or English. But to get across to your patients for purposes of history taking, advice on treatment or health education etc, you need to use the simple, lay version, unless your patient happens to be a medical (or health) person or a hypochondriac (who specializes in all kinds of medical complaints and ailments!)

Aches and Pains

While we're on the subject of complaints and ailments, why not try out the exercise below. See if you know the scientific and lay terms for the following, and check out the answers at the end of the exercise. We'll dissect out these terminologies in Update 3

English Terms	Scientific BM	Lay BM
pain		
pain in the neck		
chest pain		
epigastric pain		
abdominal pain		
bone pain		
back pain		
loin pain		
groin pain		
headache		
earache		
toothache		
muscle ache/pain		

Answers (Correct at the time of printing*)

English Terms	Scientific BM	Lay BM
pain	sakit/rasa sakit/ kesakitan	ditto
pain in the neck	sakit leher	ditto
chest pain	sakit dada	ditto
epigastric pain	sakit epigastrium	sakit ulu hati
abdominal pain	sakit abdomen	sakit perut
bone pain	sakit tulang	ditto/sengal tulang
back pain	sakit belakang	ditto
loin pain	sakit belakang/ pinggang	ditto
groin pain	sakit selangkang	sakit celah paha
headache	sakit kepala	ditto/pening kepala
earache	sakit telinga	ditto
toothache	sakit gigi	ditto
muscle ache/ pain	sengal-sengal/ sakit otot	ditto

* I have to slap up this disclaimer considering the rate at which Bahasa terminologies and spellings (not to mention pronunciations) change. Somehow, it makes the exodus of doctors leaving government service seems like 'the Setapak Crawl'.

Verdict on Performance

That wasn't painful, was it? I'm sure you can assess yourself now as to which bracket (this score, not your income) you belong to. If you've progressed from 'satisfactory' to 'good' or 'excellent' . . . ok, ok, I'll rephrase that . . . if you're made any kind of progress at all, I can presume we're on the right track. But if there's regression, maybe I should adopt a more serious approach. What do you think?

*   *   *

COMPLAINTS GALORE

Postmortem of Update 2

Update 2 demonstrated the need for doctors (as well as other professionals and academics) to be well-versed in technical as well as lay Bahasa terms. As promised, the feedback dissection of those 'painful terms' is laid out below.

Pain (as well as **ache**) takes on many versions of *sakit* such as *rasa sakit, sakit, kesakitan,* and even *sengal-sengal,* depending on the context. Occasionally, the term *nyeri* is also employed in lay usage for pain. However, for want of a better equivalent for **tender** (pain on palpation), the word *nyeri* is reserved for **tender** in the so-called *laras perubatan* (technical medical language) by defining it to mean 'tender'. If you skim through earlier translations of medical books (which you probably won't), you'll find **tender abdomen** being described as *abdomen lembut* unlike what you'll find in current translations, ie *abdomen nyeri*. *Abdomen lembut* should be interpreted as **soft abdomen** ie normal abdomen (no pathology).

Some terminologies simplify our lives greatly by being usable both ways for example: *sakit leher, sakit dada, sakit gigi* etc (the ones with *ditto* for lay BM in Update 2) can be used for both technical and lay communication . . . but not *sakit perut*. In common everyday usage, *perut* can mean stomach or abdomen. But if this dual meaning is to be maintained in *laras perubatan* (remember the problem with *kaki* for **foot** and **leg?**), the current status of poor communication will be compounded. So the term *abdomen* is adopted (for **abdomen**), and *perut* is specific for **stomach**, but when the English version (say in translation work) is **gaster**, the Bahasa equivalent is likewise **_gaster_**.

Sakit hati is another kettle of fish altogether for this (*sakit hati* ie) is a figure of speech meaning **angry** or **annoyed**. It does not refer to pain from the liver. This perhaps explains the resistance to **_hati_**, in preference for **hepar**. Otherwise we'll get medical students translating **hepatomegaly _(hepatomegali)_** to *besar hati!*

More Complaints

This month I'll give you a break . . . no terminology exercise but be prepared to hear more complaints, the kind you get to hear day in and day out in your clinic. Comments and explanations are also given where needed (tagged by asterisks). So there will be no postmortem feedback in Update 4

English Terms	*Technical BM*	*Lay BM*
fever	*demam*	ditto
pyrexia	*pireksia*	*demam*
malaise	*dedar*	ditto/*lesu/tak sedap badan*
cough	*batuk*	ditto
vomit	*muntah*	ditto

hemoptysis	*hemoptisis*	*batuk darah*
hematemesis	*hematemesis*	*muntah darah*
nausea	*mual/loya*	ditto
diarrhea	*diarea*	*cirit-birit*
constipation*	*sembelit*	ditto/*susah buang air besar/ susah berak*
dyspnea*	*dispnea*	*sesak nafas/ penat*
palpitations	*debaran*	ditto
pallor	*kepucatan*	ditto
dysuria	*disuria*	*kencing pedih/ sakit*
boil	*bisul*	ditto
ulcer	*ulser*	*luka/kudis/etc*
rash	*ruam*	ditto
pruritus	*pruritus*	*gatal-gatal*
injured	*cedera*	ditto
swollen	*bengkak*	ditto/*benjol*
fracture*	*fraktur*	*patah (tulang)*
wound	*luka*	ditto
burns*	*bakaran*	*terbakar/kena api/etc*
impotence	*impotens*	*mati pucuk/ lemah tenaga batin*
abortion	*keguguran*	ditto
pregnant	*hamil*	ditto/ *mengandung*
sterile	*mandul*	ditto

anxiety	*keresahan*	ditto/*gelisah/ semua tak kena/ etc*
headache*	*sakit kepala*	ditto/*pening kepala*
giddy*	*pening*	*kepala pusing*
blackout	*pitam*	ditto
unconscious	*tak sedar diri*	ditto
fits*	*sawan*	ditto
epilepsy*	*epilepsi*	*sawan babi*
stroke*	*strok*	*sakit/angin ahmar*
hemiplegia	*hemiplegia*	*mati sebelah*
hemiparesis	*hemiparesis*	*lemah sebelah*

Comments

Sembelit has now replaced the earlier term of *konstipasi,* when the easy way out of mere spellchange ruled *istilah* (terminology) activities. The rationale behind this move is that there is nothing technical about the term **constipation** as it is also used by lay English-speaking people. There is similar tendency towards **kepatahan** in the hope of displacing ***fraktur*** but terminology experts insist that *patah* be reserved for **broken** (bones).

Most people usually complain of **"sesak nafas"** when they get **dyspneic** but watch out for the lay Kedahans for (like most Northerners) they tend to stick to their own slang. They might complain of being **"penat"** (which most other people especially non-Kedahans interpret as **tired**) instead of sesak nafas. **Pening** may be another source of confusion for when a patient says "saya pening", s/he could be referring to either **giddiness** (correctly) or **headache** (wrongly) . . . so you have to take pains to be on the same wavelength (failing which **you** may have to take panadol five minutes later!). If you've got a splitting headache right now, it is quite understandable, but don't split yet . . . there's more to come!

Kebakaran cannot be used for **burns** as this word refers to **fire**, so **bakaran** is used instead, meaning 'effect of being burnt'.

If a mother complains of **sawan** in her baby, it implies **fits** or **thrush**. But if it is **sawan babi**, the condition is **epilepsy**.

Sakit or **angin ahmar** (lay BM for **stroke**) is not as popular as the other angins so frequently complained of, and diagnosed too! Maybe we should try to be a little more specific, while still maintaining simplicity, when we try to explain away ailments to our patients instead of dismissing them as the universal *angin* . . . . hoping perhaps the *angin* will be gone with the wind in no time.

FYI (For your info . . .)

the above list of terms on symptomatology is, of course, far from exhaustive. For those who are in a hurry to be acquainted with all the terms (at least those we have managed to compile), there is the purple book on medical terminology entitled *Istilah Perubatan, Edisi 1982* at the supercheap price of RM6.50 from university bookstores or direct from *Dewan Bahasa dan Pustaka (DBP)*. There is no guarantee, however, on its up-to-dateness, considering its age! A better move would be to wait patiently for the *Kamus Perubatan*, scheduled to hit the bookstands by the last quarter of this year! The best move, needless to say, is to be an ardent fan of this Update column!! Bye for now.

*   *   *

LET'S GET PHYSICAL

The last Update showed you how your patients might complain of their ailments (lay Bahasa) and how or what terminology you should use in the documentation of these complaints (technical Bahasa). As cautioned previously, the list was far from complete, but they should do for a start. The next logical step is to record the findings of the physical examination, which is the business of this issue of the Update.

Terms on Physical Findings

The list below attempts to give mainly the technical Bahasa terms. Since not all clinical findings need to be explained to the patient, only those deemed useful for patient information will be given their lay Bahasa equivalents. Understandably, demographic variations of lay Bahasa jargon is beyond the scope of this humble Update! Familiarization in this area would require on-site integration with the local folks for consequent (linguistic) naturalization.

English Terms	*Technical BM*	*Lay BM*
Physical Examination (Pemeriksaan Fizikal)		
inspection	*inspeksi*	*pemeriksaan*
palpation	*palpasi*	*pemeriksaan*
percussion	*perkusi*	*pemeriksaan*
auscultation	*auskultasi*	*pemeriksaan*
General Observations (Pemerhatian Umum)		
neatly attired	*berpakaian kemas*	
looks **well**	*kelihatan **sihat***	
looks **ill**	*kelihatan **sakit***	
pale	*pucat*	
anemic	*anemik*	*pucat/kurang darah*

jaundiced	ada/terdapat jaundis	sakit kuning
cyanosed	ada/terdapat sianosis	
in **pain**	pesakit **kesakitan**	
in s**hock**	terenjat/mengalami **renjatan**	
unconscious	tak sedar diri	
rational	rasional	
confused	keliru	
clubbing	penombolan	
normal	normal	biasa/baik/ normal
abnormal	abnormal	

Cardiovascular Findings (Penemuan Kardiovaskular)

pulse	nadi	
tachycardia	takikardia	
bradycardia	bradikardia	
blood pressure	tekanan darah	
heart sounds	bunyi jantung	
dual rhythm	dua rentak	
arrhythmia	aritmia	
murmur	deruan	
pansystolic	pansistolik	
apex beat	denyut apeks	
edema	edema	sembab
ascites	asites	busung
varicose veins	vena varikos	urat timbul/ kembang

Comments

The technical Bahasa equivalents for **inspection, palpation, percussion** and **auscultation** basically remain the same, with spelling change of course. **Raba** was initially suggested for **palpate** but was not widely accepted because *raba* (it is felt) bears a sexual connotation, and therefore ought to be used exclusively for cases of sexual assault such as rape. **Rasa** was likewise unsatisfactory because this word can mean **feel** as well as **taste**. **Ketuk (to knock)** for **percuss** was also knocked off the *Istilah* Register as being inaccurate. But in explaining to your patients that you're about to inspect, palpate, percuss or auscultate them, it is quite sufficient to say *"Saya nak **periksa** perut (dada, kaki, whatever) Encik"*. The main thing is that you talk to them, and non-fluency in Bahasa should not be the stumbling block, as is sometimes the case.

It is just as important to tell your patients that **everything is fine** (if it is) for example: ***"Encik tak ada apa-apa, semuanya baik"*** or ***"Semuanya biasa saja"*** or even ***"Semuanya normal"*** to the better-educated. **Normal** (like a lot of other accepted terms derived from English or Latin / Greek) is something even some academics are not familiar with, as is evident in their professional writing.

Pulse used to be *pulsus* but had of late given way to **nadi**. But **pulsus alternans** and other similar Latin terms are adopted in toto (with modified Bahasa spelling where relevant). **Finger clubbing** may be descibed as **penombolan** (from **tombol** meaning **knob**) or **pembelantanan** (from **belantan** meaning **club** or **baton**). Literalists naturally would like to promote *pembelantanan*, but pragmatists like me, prefer *penombolan* (less of a mouthful and just as accurate). Lay people use **urat** for **blood vessels** as well as **nerves**. If they have **varicose veins**, they would probably complain of "**Urat timbul**" or "**Nampak urat**" (not the same as *nampak* **aurat** with the revived mini-skirts of *Video Fashion*), and "**Tersilap urat**" if they have a **'muscle-pull'** or a **sprain** . . . . in which case they might go for an **urut (massage).**

Shock (in medicine) is popularly referred to as **renjatan**, even though some are more inclined towards **kejutan** (used commonly in engineering for **electrical shock**). Time will tell whether the distinction between the two should remain. One or two psychiatrists occasionally lament they're confused between **keliru** and **celaru**. To me, they're more or less the same . . . . **confused** (*keliru* and *celaru* ie). *Celaru* perhaps smacks of disorganisation, leading to confusion.

I guess that's it for now . . . we'll get more physical (on my terms) next month. Before I confuse you any further, **cheerio . . .** (a touch of post-Congress Irish hangover, here) and cheer up for a Happy Deepavali.

*   *   *

IT'S OUT!

What's out? The **Kamus Perubatan***lah* (**Medical Dictionary**)! What else do you think should come out after getting physical on my terms? As promised earlier, this long-awaited bible of medical terms has at last hit the bookstands, at the cheap price of RM15.00. I shall not go any further with the advertising lest Big Brother MMC (Malaysian Medical Council) summons me for a lecture on **medical ethics (*etika perubatan*)** and **advertising (*pengiklanan*)**. Suffice it to say that it is not the easiest thing in the world to get discipline experts in the deep, wide world of medicine to sit on the panel of editors (granted . . . they have more pressing things to do!) Hence the infant *Kamus* was born, not without **congenital defects (*defek kongenital*)** and inborn errors of typography. Its conception was easy but the labor was long and hard. This baby was exhausting but not exhaustive . . . the letter J carries only 23 terms! (In some ways it is simpler than Sesame Street). So please respond to it by: first of all, buying it, second of all, using it, and last of all, diagnosing the congenital defects and letting us know . . . and you'll see a brand new, improved *kamus* in the not-too-distant future. On second thought, I'll beat you to it and spot the major defects myself . . . you pick out the ones I missed! So it looks like my promise for more physical terms will have to wait. We'll do this in the next issue perhaps.

In Terms of non-Endearment

Even though the coining of new terms is governed by some guidelines, it is very difficult sometimes to agree on them. Therefore in coming up with the *Kamus Perubatan*, (which is no mean feat), these gray areas manifest in the form of inconsistencies and controversies. Some of these are highlighted below under the following categories:

Lay versus Scientific

The medical profession is sometimes pressured into accepting terms which are okay at the lay and school levels, but not acceptable for higher education or the profession. For example, the *Kamus Perubatan* advocates the following lay terms rather than the preferred technical or scientific ones (in brackets):

auricle	*daun telinga* **(aurikel)**
clavicle	*tulang selangka* **(klavikel)**
scapula	*tulang belikat* **(skapula)**
fontanel	*ubun-ubun* **(fontanel)**
uterus	*rahim* **(uterus)**
pudendum	*kemaluan* **(pudendum)**
relapse	*kambuh* **(relaps)**
recrudescence	*bentan* **(rekrudesens)**

Inappropriate or Inaccurate

I find the following terms unacceptable but the younger generation may not agree with me as they have the benefit of Malay-medium education which I lack. It would be nice to get feedback on these terms from you guys who are (supposed to be) already using them in your professional writing! The preferred terms and some comments are given in brackets.

simple goiter	*goiter ringkas* (**goiter simpel**. 'Simple fruits' are referred to as *buah ringkas* in school, hence, *goiter ringkas!)*
complicated fracture	*fraktur rumit* (***fraktur terkomplikasi?*** This one is truly *rumit* / complex).
glucose	*glukosa* (***glukos**. Ironically, glukos is considered OK for lay usage. Other similar terms include **dekstrosa** for **dextrose**, **fluorida** for **fluoride**, **amina** for **amine** and so on).
induction	***pengaruhan (induksi.** **Pengaruhan** may lead to confusion in some context because it is better known to mean **'influence'**).
plantar flexion	*fleksi kaki* (***fleksi plantar**. **Dorsiflexion**, however, is listed as **dorsifleksi**).
fluorescence	*pendarfluor* (***fluoresens**. The prefix 'pen- ' suggests a 'doer' such as **penimbal** for **buffer** but fluorescence does not belong to this category).

| precursor | *pelopor* (**prakursor. Pelopor**, meaning **pioneer**, was expanded in concept to avoid using *prakursor*, the term which makes more sense.) |

Inconsistent

The guidelines postulate that Latin or Greek terms accepted in toto in English/American usage should also be given the same treatment, with spellchange according to the Bahasa spelling system. Unfortunately a few of such terms were overlooked, but not to worry . . . the correct ones are given in brackets below:

delirium tremens	*racauan tremens* **(delirium tremens).**
otitis external/internal	*otitis luaran / dalaman* **(otitis external/internal**. Otitis media, however, is not listed).
paralysis agitans	*kelumpuhan agitans* **(paralisis agitans).**

Simply Unacceptable

The following words (to name a few) are not acceptable by some lecturers as they claim the word is either alien or too crude for proper usage:

urine   *(air) kencing* (The preferred term, at least by many medical lecturers, is **urin** as they think **kencing** is too crude. Well . . . "they ain't heard nuthin' yet" as the Yanks would say. Read on and you'll see what I mean!).

feces   **tinja.** (This is the alien one, a migrant term from Indonesia which, according to some, should be reserved for the **stool of a Ninja!** Others prefer **najis** but this is frowned upon as a religious term referring to any **bodily excretions**. Still others advocate **feses** but was rejected as bull, but the prize went to DBP (*Dewan Bahasa dan Pustaka*) who initially wanted **tahi** which was truly [and literally] **shit**. Most people find *tahi* rather shitty, [pardon the term] but really, it is **the** common word used in Kedah and perhaps the other northern states too. Let's take another look at *kencing*—it doesn't sound too crude now does it?).

liver	*hati* (**hepar**). **Hati**, being a **figurative** word in Bahasa, is often confused for **heart** (**jantung**) for example: **jantung hati** is **sweetheart** or a **loved one.** **Sakit hati** is again a figurative expression, meaning **annoyed** or **jealous** (**iri hati**). Therefore, in a medical (especially psychiatric) scenario, we can never be sure whether a patient is annoyed or jealous of someone or he has **liver pain** (pain from liver diseases).

Too much of a mouthful

Many *Bahasa* editors recommended terms which are simply unpronounceable by the average medical person, whose tongue has been fixated by English education from primary school through tertiary and postgraduate training, and finally lifelong learning via CME (Continuing Medical Education). Try rolling your tongue with these:

inbreeding	*pembiakbakaan dalam* (any offers??)
opsonic index	*indeks pengopsoninan* (**indeks opsonik**)
uterine inertia	*kelengaian uterus* (**inertia uterus**)

viable	*berdaya hidup (**viable***. *Berdaya hidup* is the definition rather than a term)

These goof-ups might have been avoided if the people involved in the formulation of **'Terminology Guidelines'** were more appreciative of consumer factors such as acceptability and practicality. But whatever the shortcomings, the *Kamus Perubatan* is yet another feather in the cap of *Bahasa* Medical Terminologists and DBP. (The first feather was the **Istilah Perubatan**). Your views and suggestions would go a long way in finetuning the medical language in *Bahasa Malaysia*. **Selamat membeli kamus!**

* See Update 7: Spellbound by Spellchange

*   *   *

LET'S GET MORE PHYSICAL

More 'Physical Terms'

Now that the *Kamus Perubatan* (Update 5: It's Out!) is out of the way, we can carry on where we left off in Update 4 to talk about more physical terms. As in Update 4, the terms are listed in mainly technical Bahasa, and only those deemed useful for patient information are given their lay Bahasa equivalents (in brackets) in the list. Some terms, of course, cannot strictly be classified as technical or lay in nature—they serve both types of communicators equally well.

English	**Bahasa Malaysia**

Respiratory Findings (Penemuan Pernafasan)

English	Bahasa Malaysia
lungs	*peparu / paru-paru*
bronchus	*bronkus*
lobe	*lobus*
windpipe	*salur udara*
trachea	*trakea (salur udara)*
deviated (trachea)	*teranjak*
air entry	*masukan udara*
tachypneic	*takipneik*
crepitations	*krepitasi*
rhonchi	*ronkus*
wheeze	*weez*
resonance	*resonans*
dull (on percussion)	*?????* (I'm not so bright on this one!)

Alimentary Findings (Penemuan Alimentari)

English	Bahasa Malaysia
abdomen	*abdomen (perut)*
hypochondrium	*hipokondrium*
epigastrium	*epigastrium (ulu hati)*
lumbar region/flank	*kawasan lumbar*
umbilical region	*kawasan umbilikus (kawasan pusat)*
right iliac fossa	*fosa ilium kanan*

hypogastrium	*hipogastrium*
umbilicus	*umbilikus (pusat)*
anterior superior iliac spine	*spina ilium superior anterior*
soft (abdomen)	*lembut (abdomen)*
tender	*nyeri*
rebound tenderness	*nyeri pantulan ('pantulan' is still being debated—the culprit here being 'rebound')*
shifting dullness	*????? bergerak (Even our linguists are stumped by 'dullness')*
distension	*distensi (buncit)*
distended	*buncit*
ascites	*asites (busung/buncit perut)*
rigid	*tegang*
guarded	*mendinding (tegang/keras)*
borborygmi	*borborigmi (bunyi perut)*
bowel sounds	*bunyi usus*
peristaltic waves	*gerak peristalsis*
palpable masses	*jisim terpalpat*
hepatomegaly	*hepatomegali*
splenomegaly	*splenomegali*
hepatosplenomegaly	*hepatosplenomegali*
hernia	*hernia (burut)*
femoral/inguinal hernia	*hernia femoral/inguinal*

direct/indirect hernia	*hernia langsung/tak langsung*
hemorrhoids	*hemoroid*
piles	*buasir*
caput medusae	*kaput medusa*
halithosis	*halitosis (nafas berbau)*

Discussion

Respiratory Terms

Terms on physical findings of the respiratory system are notorious for bringing on respiratory distress among terminologists on account of the paucity of equivalents in *Bahasa Malaysia*. As can be seen from the list, there are no popular terms that you can use to explain respiratory sounds like **crepitations, rhonchi** and **wheeze** to your patients. We have scoured various ancient *kamuses* until we turned **dyspneic *(dispneik)*,** we have yet to stumble upon Bahasa words for descriptive English terms like **dull** (on percussion), let alone **stony dullness.** The prospects are dull indeed for this part of the body to be Malaysianized! By the way, the term for **lung(s)** is ***peparu*** or ***paru-paru***. There is no such thing as ***paru***, which is concocted by some for (one) lung, just as paru-paru is mistaken for the two (lungs).

Abdominal / Alimentary Terms

Major anatomical zones and landmarks have to be familiarized with before you can document your findings. **Hypochondrium, epigastrium, lumbar, umbilical, iliac fossa, hypogastrium** and **anterior superior iliac spine (ASIS)** are all very technical-sounding, and are therefore maintained as such in *Bahasa* with mere spellchange.

Abdomen *(abdomen)*, **soft** *(lembut)*, **tender** *(nyeri)* and **ascites** *(asites)* had already been discussed in previous Updates. Unfortunately the *Bahasa* equivalent for **rebound** (tenderness) is still unknown to most of us in the *Istilah* (Terminology) department. For **rebound tenderness**, I am suggesting here that we use *nyeri pantulan* which is not spot-on but will have to do for now until we coin up something more succint. Abdominal **guarding** is described as *mendinding* (to wall up), ie 'to guard' or 'to protect'.

Distensi is maintained for **distension** in favor over *kembung* **(flatulence)** which is merely a specific type/cause of distension. Other causes of distension can be **abdominal masses** *(jisim abdomen)*. Here *jisim* is used instead of *massa* because **massa** is reserved 'for the **masses'** for example: *media massa* **(mass media)** or *rawatan massa* **(mass therapy)**. The other causes for distension viz **splenomegaly, hepatomegaly** and **hepatosplenomegaly** are highly technical terms using the Latin suffix '-megaly'. Such Anglicized technical terms (especially with Latin or Greek derivatives) are the easiest to translate—they remain the same, except for spelling, as mentioned above.

Some linguistic purists may pressure us to use *bunyi usus* for **borborygmi**, but the general practice is to maintain the technical-versus-lay status, ie lay for lay and likewise for technical. Thus, we insist on *borborigmi* for **borborygmi** and *bunyi usus* for **bowel sounds.** The same can be said for **trachea** vs **windpipe** (*trakea* vs *salur udara*), **hemorrhoids** vs **piles** (*hemoroid* vs *buasir*), and *hernia* vs *burut*. I suppose other alternatives for **gerak peristalsis** (**peristaltic waves**) can be *ombak peristalsis* (to please the literalists) or *gelombang peristalsis* (for lovers of the long . . . and winded!), but not *gerakan peristalsis* (too political!).

Unlike the respiratory system, the alimentary tract is quite elementary and *Bahasa*-friendly. In fact so friendly that we have idiomatic expressions (whispering words of wisdom) using pathological body parts such as *"Tiada **burut**, diampu-ampu"*. ("Why wear a truss when you don't have a **hernia**?"). Popular terms for this condition are also aplenty; these include **sakit pasang-pasang** (which may also refer to **hydrocele**), **sakit ulur-ulur** (**not ular-ular**, please) and **sakit bodek** which may well define the new, yet-to-be-documented syndrome in the *SSB*! (By the way, the *SSB* or *Sistem Saraan Baru* or New Remuneration System for employees in the Malaysian public service is fondly known as *"Saya Sayang Bos"* or "I Love Boss". *Bodek* (apple polish) the boss and you've got yourself a supersonic career pathway. Of course this is not true of all bosses!

I guess that's it for now. May I wish all Muslim *istilah* lovers ***"Selamat Berpuasa"*. (Happy Fasting).** 'Tis again the season for Ramadhan-inspired gastritis!

*　　*　　*

UPDATE 7

SPELLBOUND BY SPELLCHANGE

First and foremost, let me point out with a thousand apologies, that the *Bahasa* term **'viabel'** in "Update 5" was misspelt (as **'viable'**—in the monthly MMA newsletter) by not being given the spellchange treatment! Spelling errors are rampant nowadays where English terms are spelt the *Bahasa* way and vice versa. Such in the price of technical bilingualism . . . and sheer carelessness or ignorance. Even though I have reminded you *ad nauseam* in previous updates about spellchange when translating a technical term from English to *Bahasa Malaysia*, I have yet to discuss the *Bahasa* Spelling Guidelines. However, I'm sure most of you have figured out a good deal already as, by and large, *Bahasa* is a relatively simple language with a logical spelling system that appreciates the sense of sound. And when the vocabulary concerns terms which are derived from the already familiar language of English, the whole process of English-*Bahasa* conversion becomes a breeze.

Some Guidelines in Medical Bahasa Spelling

I have to emphasize (so you'll not be misguided) that these guidelines I'm about to discuss refer to only technical terms. In this particular Update, I'm not concerned with linguistic crimes like that of Dr X who apologized in court *"Maaf, saya **liwat** sebab . . .".* ("Sorry, I **sodomized** because . . .") when he should have said *"Maaf, saya **lewat** sebab . . . .".* (But I really do not recommend Dr X to be struck off the Register for linguistic negligence . . . . unless of course, there's no mistake in his apology!) For the sake of simplicity and my philosophy of telling it like it is, I shall discuss the spelling guide under 5 headings namely: 1) Vowels 2) Consonants 3) Endings 4) Special Names and 5) Status Ambiguous.

1) Vowels

With some exceptions, most vowels remain unchanged in Bahasa terms.

Examples include:

lateral	*lateral* (not leteral)
migraine	*migrain* (not migren)
aorta	*aorta*
autonomic	*autonomik* (not '*otonomik*' as 'oto-' pertains to the ear)
analgesia	analgesia (not analgisia)
pineal	*pineal* (but 'ear' is not 'ear', it is '*telinga*')
protein	*protein* (not *protin*)
eosinophilia	*eosinofilia* (not *iosinofilia*)
leukemia	*leukemia* (not *liukemia*)
pleura	*pleura* (not *plura*)
histology	*histologi*
iatrogenic	*iatrogenik*
species	*spesies* (not *spesis*)
angiitis	*angiitis* (not *angitis*)
iodine	*iodin* (not *aidin*)
myocardium	*miokardium*
zona pellucida	*zona pelusida*
steroid	*steroid*
zoonosis	*zoonosis* (not *zunosis*)
ulcer	*ulser* (not *alser*)
dualism	*dualisme*
duodenum	*duodenum*

Exceptions include:

jo<u>u</u>rnal	*j<u>u</u>rnal*
<u>oe</u>sophagus	*<u>e</u>sofagus* (however you can forget about this exception by thinking American, like what I've been doing all along. And if you've bought the *Kamus Perubatan* like I suggested, you would have noticed that the English entries in the *Kamus* are all American. This way, the English entry in this case becomes 'esophagus' and the 'oe' exception is nullified!)
an<u>ae</u>mia	*an<u>e</u>mia* (same argument as above)

Note:

<u>ae</u>robic	*<u>ae</u>robik* (You can't Americanize this as even the Americans do not take their usual shortcuts with this word. This is because the **'ae'** here means **'air'** and this spelling is therefore in line with the spelling system.)
homolog<u>ue</u>	*homolog* (The terminal **'ue'** has no vocal role and is therefore dropped.)

2) Consonants

a) Most consonants are maintained and are only changed to be phonetically sensible.

Examples:

<u>c</u>arbon	<u>k</u>arbon
s<u>ch</u>izophrenia	s<u>k</u>izofrenia
<u>cy</u>stitis	<u>si</u>stitis
s<u>c</u>iatica	siatika (The silent 'c' is omitted but the 'c' in **fascia** and its derivatives are maintained to avoid confusion between the facially-derived **fasiorafi** and the fascially-derived **fas<u>c</u>iorafi**).
<u>rh</u>initis	<u>r</u>initis
<u>ph</u>armacy	farmasi
<u>th</u>erapy	terapi (much to the annoyance of some pharmacologists as they were often tricked into saying **'ter-api'** in the early days of istilah development.)
as<u>th</u>ma	asma (By spelling rule it should be astma but **asma** was so well-established and accepted . . . anyway what's another exception?)

equine	*ekuin* (Obviously **Q fever** is **demam Q** . . . . which is one of the almost non-existent 'Q' in Bahasa vocabulary)
tetralogy	*tetralogi* (to give 'y' the sound of 'i')

Exceptions include:

xanthoma	*xantoma* (not *zantoma*)
psychiatry	*psikiatri* (not *saikiatri* or even *sakaitri*)

b) **Consonant couples** (unlike double vowels) are reduced to singles unless misleading.

Examples:

allele	*alel*
mammary glands	*kelenjar mamari* (It used to be *kelenjar mama* but several papas protested as they too are proud owners of these glands . . . . trust the gents to make mountains out of molehills).

Exceptions include:

ammonia	*ammonia* (A single 'm' if it were *amonia* gives the visual

	impact of a prefix to the first 'a' meaning 'without', thus misleading fresh students and stale lecturers . . . or so the argument goes!)
re<u>nn</u>in	*re<u>nn</u>in* (Another *renin* already exists).
se<u>rr</u>atus anterior	*se<u>rr</u>atus anterior* (A single 'r' would give seratus or 100 anteriors).
va<u>cc</u>ine	*va<u>ks</u>in* (to give the Bahasa sense of sound which *'vacin'* fails to do).

3) Endings

Some endings of terms are subject to the process of addition, deletion, substitution or transposition:

a) **Substitution:**

Certain words ending with -**tion** or -**sion** are converted to *Bahasa* by substituting them with -*si*. (Please note that I said 'certain' because this leeway is only for those words which become very troublesome if we use proper *Bahasa* **Example:** *koagulasi* is more manageable than *pengkoagulasian* but **immunisation** is *pengimunan* not *imunisasi* like in the good old days, when even *televisi* was visually acceptable).

Examples:

hallucina<u>tion</u>	*halusina<u>si</u>*
delu<u>sion</u>	*delu<u>si</u>* (easy huh!)

b) **Addition:**

Certain words ending with -erm, -asm, -ism are given an extra 'a' or 'e'.

Examples:

ectoderm	*ektoderm<u>a</u>*
sperm	*sperm<u>a</u>*
protoplasm	*protoplasm<u>a</u>* ('a' for something tangible)
orgasm	*orgasm<u>e</u>* ('e' for abstract non-tangibles like behavior, experience, ideology, etc)
organism	*organism<u>a</u>* (tangible)
sadism	*sadism<u>e</u>* (non-tangible)

c) **Deletion:**

The terminal **'e'** of most words are **deleted**, with or without substitution.

Examples:

sulphat_e_	*sulfat*
spirochet_e_	*spiroket*
lymphocyt_e_	*limfosit*
relaps_e_	*relaps*
tissu_e_	*tisu*
atmospher_e_	*atmosfera* (not *atmosfer*)
spor_e_	*spora* (not *spor*)
fluorid_e_	*fluorida* (not *fluorid*)

Exceptions include:

amilas_e_	*amylase.* (As you have guessed, we can't afford to change the terminal '-ase' to '-as' for enzymes unless we want to transform **lipase** to a **cockroach *(lipas).***
hydrocel_e_	*hidrosele* (the terminal 'e' is maintained to avoid -***sel*** which gives the visual impression of **cell**)
systole / diastole	*sistole / diastole*

d) **Transposition:**

In some words, the terminal **'le'** after a consonant are transposed to **'el'**.

Examples:

viab<u>le</u>   *viab<u>el</u>*

vesic<u>le</u>   *vesik<u>el</u>*

4) Special Names

a) **Drug Names**

To avoid confusion which might lead to grave side effects such as death, drug names are maintained in toto except that in *Bahasa*, the first letters are capitalized.

Examples:

penicillin G   <u>P</u>enicillin G (but the **penicillin** group of antibiotics is spelt ***penisilin***, again making pharmacologists very melancholy)

ampicillin   <u>A</u>mpicillin (not *ampisilin*)

b) **Organisms and Infections**

Just as for drugs, groups of specific organisms and the infections they cause are spelt *Bahasa*-style but names of species or the genera are maintained in toto.

Examples:

Streptococcus sp	*Streptococcus sp* (but the group of **streptococci** are spelt ***streptokokus*** in the singular form . . . . you've guessed it—melancholic microbiologists).
Plasmodium vivax	*Plasmodium vivax*
to<u>x</u>oplasmosis	*to<u>ks</u>oplasmosis* (usual spellchange)

5) Status Ambiguous

a) You now know that names of species or genera (for example: *Salmonella* sp) are maintained in toto but the infections they cause are modified, spellingwise (for example: ***salmonelosis***). However, it is still being debated whether **S. typhi** should cause **salmonelosis typhi** or **salmonelosis tifi**. The same argument rages between proponents of ***malaria vivax*** and those of ***malaria vivaks***. And no one is sure whether **<u>shigellosis</u>** should be **_shigelosis_** or **_sygelosis_** (compare the current **_skuasy_** with the old **_skuash_** for **squash**).

b) A cold war is also brewing underground among champions of **_glukos_** vs **_glukosa, amin_** vs **_amina, logik_** vs **_lojik, agen_** vs **_ejen,_** _Baku_ vs non-_Baku_ . . . with no clear truce in sight. This keeps us all spell-bound by the current spelling system. Nevertheless, it provides many opportunities for meetings and academic discussions.

As far as I am concerned, it is probably best if we don't mess around with the _Baku_ issue (of pronouncing every letter to the letter), unless we enjoy saying **'pee-see-core-law-ghee'** (for **psikologi**). The other reason is that my user-friendly phonetics might earn me the title of phoney phonetician! Frankly, I don't think MMC can handle one more phoney at the moment . . . what with bogus cosmetic surgeons cutting loose in the city! Till next month, **_selamat menyambut Hari Wesak_** (Happy Wesak Day).

*   *   *

UPDATE 8

BAHASA AID FOR AIDS

I heard from the MMA Grapevine that the public forum for this year's AGM had plenty to do with AIDS, hence the topic for this Update. Some quarters translate the **Aquired Immunodeficiency Syndrome** as *Sindrom Kurang Upaya Daya Tahan*. This may be good enough for the lay public but not quite adequate for the profession, as the keyword 'acquired' is ignored. The truth is however, whether you correctly call it *'**Sindrom Kurang Imun <u>Perolehan</u>**'* or not, no one will understand you unless you refer to it as simply 'AIDS' (not SKIP). And if I may expose my true puritanical self, I'd say the naked truth is that this modern curse would not plague us today if we *Homo sapiens* (including *Homo homos*) were to think twice before monkeying around with just about anybody . . . (African leaf monkeys, you take note!) The demand for a **cure *(penyembuhan)*** and a **vaccine *(vaksin)*** will only drain the nation's resources, as long as the thrust of education is still to condomize society and sterilize syringes. OK, enough preaching . . . let's get on with the aid.

AIDS Glossary

The Virus and Transmission	*(Virus dan Penularan)*
Human Immunodeficiency Virus (HIV)	*Virus Imunodefisiensi Manusia* (HIV not VIM, internationally used acronyms are maintained)
high risk groups	*golongan risiko tinggi* (not *gulungan*)
sexual intercourse	*persetubuhan*
homosexual	*homoseks*

hemophiliac	*hemofiliak* (or *pesakit hemofilia*)
factor VIII preparations	*sediaan faktor VIII*
drug addict	*penagih dadah*
prostitute	*pelacur*
blood transfusion	*transfusi darah* (*pemindahan darah* is a lay term)
transplacental	*transplasenta*
syringe	*picagari*
intravenous	*intravena*
infected body fluids	*cecair tubuh terinfeksi*

Clinical Manifestations and Disease States	**(Manifestasi Klinikal dan Tahap Penyakit)**
HIV carrier	*pembawa HIV*
AIDS related complex (ARC)	*Kompleks Kaitan AIDS* (ARC not KKA)
opportunistic infections	*infeksi oportunis*
Pneumocystis pneumonia (PCP)	*pneumonia Pneumocystis* (PCP)
oral candidiasis	*kandidiasis oral*
hairy leukoplakia	*leukoplakia berbulu (?)*
chronic diarrhea	*diarea kronik*
cryptosporidiosis	*kriptosporidiosis*
isosporiasis	*isosporiasis*
anal herpes	*herpes anus*
subacute encephalitis	*ensefalitis subakut*

cryptococcal meningitis	*meningitis kriptokokus*
cerebral toxoplasmosis	*toksoplasmosis serebral*
persistent generalized	*limfadenopati*
lymphadenopathy (PGL)	*menyeluruh persisten*
	(PGL not LMP)
infectious mononucleosis	*mononukleosis berjangkit*
Kaposi's sarcoma	*sarcoma Kaposi*
Non-Hodgkin's lymphoma	*limfoma bukan Hodgkin*
anxiety	*keresahan*

Anti-HIV Test	**(Ujian Anti-HIV)**
HIV antibody test	*ujian antibodi HIV*
T-lymphocyte test	*ujian limfosit-T*
Western blot assay	*asai 'Western blot'*
test accuracy	*ketepatan ujian*
implications	*implikasi*

Controling the Spread	**(Mengawal Perebakan)**
education campaigns	*kempen pendidikan*
target groups	*golongan sasaran*
epidemiological investigations	*siasatan epidemiologi*
blood screening	*penyaringan darah*
diagnosis of HIV infections/AIDS	*pendiagnosan infeksi HIV/AIDS*

patient management	*pengendalian* (not *pengurusan*) *pesakit*
disinfection	*disinfeksi* (NOT *nyahinfeksi!*)
report and evaluation	*laporan* (not *lapuran*) *dan penilaian*
isolation	*pengasingan/pemencilan*
counseling	*kaunseling*
emotional support	*sokongan emosi*
safe sex	*seks selamat*
condom	*kondom*
treatment	*rawatan*
medication	*pengubatan*
immune modulators	*modulator imun*
reverse transcriptase inhibitors	*perencat transkriptase berbalik*
zidovudine (AZT)	**Zidovudine* (AZT) **(*See footnote)**
isoprinosine	**Isoprinosine* **(*See footnote)**
interferon	*Interferon*
interleukin-2	*Interleukin-2*
cytotoxic drugs	*dadah sitotoksik*
cosmetic radiotherapy	*radioterapi kosmetik*
marrow transplant	*transplantasi sumsum*

* *(Drug names in Bahasa begin with capital letters)*

Discussion

Ever since we went metric, we all know that a gram of **prevention** *(pencegahan)* is worth a kilo of cure but **safe sex** is bound to illicit multiple interpretations. For a start, there is probably no such thing as safe sex anymore except no-sex or abstinence, hence the promotion of **'safer sex'** *(seks yang lebih selamat)* in a recent write-up on sex guidelines in a British Medical Association publication. Apart from discouraging people from having sex outside a regular relationship, several 'safer sex' strategies such as solo sex or **masturbation** *(merancap)* are mentioned in the booklet for both the straight and the kinky. Supercondoms are advocated for **gays** (*pondan* or colloquially, *'Mak Nyah'* who should not be equated with *peria* **(guys)** as they are far from *ria* / happy once AIDS-stricken). The global philosophy seems to be: if you can't fight those **urges** *(desakan)* a-rising from **hormonal surges** *(terpaan hormon)* as you are bounding with adolescent energy, you might as well get smart and subscribe to condoms till kingdom come.

Condom advertisers *(pengiklan kondom)* claim that we can stop the **killer** *(pembunuh)* from spreading further by advising us to: 1) Lead a **healthy lifestyle**

(gaya hidup yang sihat) 2) Never share needles and syringes . . . (it used to be "stay away from drugs") 3) Avoid promiscuous behavior (good) . . . . and then contradict themselves with a turnaround extolling the **prophylactic virtues *(kebaikan profilaksis)*** of these rubber stockings if you prefer a 'heaty' lifestyle! It is thus hard to envision their effectiveness in AIDS **control *(kawalan)*** in the long run, but more use of condoms (and use of more condoms) sure is a boost to the rubber industry! Use of more condoms is also a surefire prophylaxis (claim some quarters), because by the time the second condom is on, the fire is off! If condom use must be advised, it has to be done explicitly to prevent hot-but-dull Don Juans from donning **gloves *(sarung getah)*** instead. The moral here is: call a condom a *kondom,* not *sarung getah!*

While some people still enjoy bed-hopping despite the AIDS scare, a few are stricken with another version of AIDS which is bandied about as the 'AIDS Induced Distress Syndrome', and suffer from **anxiety *(keresahan),* insomnia *(insomnia),* nightmares *(mengigau),* night sweats *(peluh malam)*** etc. These few include those who had been sneaking behind their wives' backs to forbidden garden-of-Edens, innocent wives of playful husbands (and vice versa maybe), and patients who had received **blood transfusions** *(transfusi darah).* These unfortunates would love to rap Bobby McFarren for advising them "Don't worry, be happy" at a time like this.

In Malaysia, the AIDS scourge is beginning to take its toll, as evidenced by rising **morbidity *(morbiditi)*** and **mortality *(mortaliti).*** There may soon be a public cry for resettlement of AIDS patients and HIV carriers in some faraway colony, like modern day lepers. (Maybe they can live on HIV Island in HIV condos, a few cynics are bound to suggest). This stems partly from the non-compassion of a not-so-caring society and partly from the various **myths *(mitos)*** clouding the AIDS issue such as its possible transmission via verbal intercourse at close proximity. The fact is even **French kissing *(kucupan Perancis?)*** involving normal mouths has been cleared by the Italians as a non-transmitter. But then what do bottom-pinchers know about kissing? To drive the point home about AIDS transmission: verbal intercourse—no, oral intercourse—yes! Celebate—no, celebrate—maybe, depending on mode of celebration.

With not a cure and a vaccine in sight, some people may resort to **alternative medicine *(perubatan*** *alternatif)* which includes **hypnotherapy *(hipnoterapi),* acupuncture *(akupunktur),* herbalism *(herbalisme)* and homeopathy *(homeopati).*** This leaves many doors wide open to quackery (ushering the return of 'Dr Zainal' and associates) . . . and there is nothing much the medical profesion can do as it does not have the answer either.

Until next month, **happy updating** . . . it's safer than dating!

*   *   *

KUIZRIA BAHASA MALAYSIA

Many moons have passed since you last had a quiz! And it's good to take stock of things once in a while to see how we're progressing. This quiz is meant to test your application of the tricks of the trade learnt from two previous Updates: Scientific versus Lay and Spellbound by Spellchange. Once done, check out the answers and feedback comments at the end! More input will be given in the next Update on the rules of translating terms comprising two or more words.

Now let's see what you can do with the following 20 questions . . . (I'm hearing cheeky answers already!)

Instructions:

Select the **<u>best</u> Bahasa Malaysia equivalent** from A-D for the following terms:

1 drug

    A   *ubat*

    B   *dadih*

    C   *dadah*

    D   *najis dadah*

2 biceps

    A   *bisep*

    B   *biseps*

    C   *baiseps*

    D   *otot dua kepala*

3 hookworm

    A   *cacing kail*

    B   *cacing kerawit*

C   *cacing kait*

D   *cacing rambo*

4   autoantibody

A   *antibodi kendiri*

B   *swa-antibodi*

C   *bodi-anti-auto*

D   *autoantibodi*

5   anxiety

A   *anzieti*

B   *keresahan*

C   *kegelisahan*

D   *kerisauan*

6   diplococcus

A   *kokus duaan*

B   *dwikokus*

C   *diplokokus*

D   *diplococcus*

7   endoscopy

A   *pandangan dalam*

B   *skop dalaman*

C   *endoskopi*

D   *tinjau di dalam*

8   neonate

A   *neonat*

B   *nionet*

C   *neonatum*

D   *bayi sebulan*

9   leg

A   *kaki*

B   *kaki bawah*

C   *tungkai*

D   *anggota bawah*

10 blood vessel

A   *pembuluh darah*

B   *saluran darah*

C *arteri*

D *vena*

11 midstream urine

A *urin midstrim*

B *kencing tengah sungai*

C *(air) kencing tengah mengalir*

D *(air) kencing aliran tengah*

12 acute arthritis

A *sendi comel*

B *radang sendi*

C *arteritis akut*

D *artritis akut*

13 automatic bar

A *palang automatik*

B *automatik palang*

C *palang otomatik*

D *palang berotomatik*

14 local anesthesia

A *anestesia tempatan*

B *anestesia setempat*

C *pelali tempatan*

D *bius setempat*

15 clinical examination

A *pemeriksaan kelinikel*

B *pemeriksaan klinikal*

C *pemeriksaan kelinik*

D *pemeriksaan klinik*

16 status asthmaticus

A *status asma*

B *taraf asma*

C *asma berstatus*

D *status asmatikus*

17 collapsing pulse

A *pulsus mengkolaps*

B *pulsus runtuh*

C   *nadi kolaps*

D   *nadi melenyap*

18 common cold

A   *selemo*

B   *selesma*

C   *selsema*

D   *selesema*

19 grand mal epilepsy

A   *sawan babi*

B   *sawan besar-besaran*

C   *epilepsi mal grand*

D   *epilepsi grand mal*

20 sympathetic nervous system

A   *sistema nervorum simpatikum*

B   *sistem saraf simpatetik*

C   *sistem saraf simpati*

D   *sistem saraf bersimpati*

Answers

1 drug = *dadah* (C)

A *ubat* (lay term, use this when talking with patients)

B *dadih* (yogurt)

D *najis dadah* (emotional term to denote **'filth'** / **najis**)

2 biceps = *biseps* (B)

A *bisep* (the terminal 's' should not be dropped, as in ambulans)

C *baiseps* (wrong spelling)

D *otot dua kepala* (a partial definition, not a term)

3 hookworm = *cacing kait* (C)

A *cacing kail* (not a recognized term, even though **kail** can also mean **hook**)

B *cacing kerawit* (you've met this **pinworm** / Enterobius before)

D *cacing rambo* (this is one macho worm; would the real *cacing **rambu*** / Trichuris please stand up? . . or crawl up?)

4   autoantibody = *autoantibodi* (D)

A   *antibodi kendiri* (even as definition, the concept is wrong)

B   *swa-antibodi* (**swa** is sometimes used for **self**, not 'auto')

C   *bodi-anti-auto* (this would be correct if 'autoantibody' were three separate words)

5   anxiety = *keresahan* (B)

A   *anzieti* (previous term when any term goes, now obsolete)

C   *kegelisahan* (more like **restlessness**)

D   *kerisauan* (**worries**)

6   diplococcus = diplokokus (C)

A   *kokus duaan* (a description, not a term)

B   *dwikokus* (getting warm, but still not acceptable)

D   *diplococcus* (spellchange for the group name)

7   endoscopy = *endoskopi* (C)

A   *pandangan dalam* (hazy explanation, may mean **penetrating look**)

    B   *skop dalaman* (technical terms need only spellchange treatment,

       Example: *mikroskop*, not *'skop mikro'*)

    D   tinjau di dalam (an explanation, good for lay usage)

8 neonate = *neonat* (A)

    B   *nionet* (wrong spelling)

    C   *neonatum* (no such '-tum', even for Latin babies!)

    D   *bayi sebulan* (definition, not the term)

9 leg = *tungkai* (C)

    A   *kaki* (do you get that 'deja foot' feeling?)

    B   *kaki bawah* (lower foot?)

    D   *anggota bawah* (lower limb, which is more than a leg)

10 blood vessel = *pembuluh darah* (A)

    B   *saluran darah* (acceptable but not the best; *saluran* = **channel**)

    C   *arteri* (a specific type of blood vessel)

    D   *vena* (another type of blood vessel)

11 midstream urine (MSU) = *(air) kencing aliran tengah* (D)

   A   *urin midstrim* (*urin* is popular but not acceptable by DBP; *midstrim* is a lazy way out, as was the case with *anzieti*)

   B   *kencing tengah sungai* (literal translation . . . still, it's quite possible to collect MSU in the middle of a river)

   C   *(air) kencing tengah mengalir* (the urine is flowing)

12 acute arthritis = *artritis akut* (D)

   A   *sendi comel* (how **cute**)

   B   *radang sendi* (incomplete description but good enough for lay usage)

   C   *arteritis akut* (check out the 'e' and chuck it out! Trick question, huh?)

13 automatic bar = *palang automatik* (A)

   B   *automatik palang* (wrong sequence)

   C   *palang otomatik* (wrong spelling)

   D   *palang berotomatik* (prefix abuse, on top of wrong spelling)

14 local anesthesia = *anestesia setempat* (B)

A *anestesia tempatan* (**tempatan** is **local** in the geographical context)

C *pelali tempatan* (**pelali** is a lay term meaning something to **numb** pain sensation)

D *bius setempat* (**bius** is the lay term for **anesthesia**)

15 clinical examination = *pemeriksaan klinikal* (B)

A *pemeriksaan kelinikel* (a common misspelling)

C *pemeriksaan kelinik* (kelinik is wrong spelling, wrong word)

D *pemeriksaan klinik* (examination of clinics)

16 status asthmaticus = *status asmatikus* (D)

A *status asma* (different meaning)

B *taraf asma* (gives same meaning as A)

C *asma berstatus* (completely nonsensical . . . asthma with a status!)

17 collapsing pulse = *nadi melenyap* (D)

A *pulsus mengkolaps* (was used, once upon a time)

B *pulsus runtuh* (**runtuh** applies to **collapsed buildings** or other structural erections)

C *nadi kolaps* (now obsolete)

18 common cold = *selesema* (D)

A *selemo* (Negri version, pronounced 'sir-lair-more')

B *selesma* (one 'e' is missing)

C *selsema* (I used to think this was correct . . . I'll be damned if DBP's Spelling Register had a typographical error!)

19 grand mal epilepsy = *epilepsi grand mal* (D)

A *sawan babi* (sometimes used by lay people for **epilepsy**)

B *sawan besar-besaran* (**besar-besaran** is **grand** in a **lavish** sense)

C *epilepsi mal grand* (wrong sequence)

20 sympathetic nervous system = **sistem saraf simpatetik (B)**

A *sistema nervorum simpatikum* (equivalent of Latin version. Generally, the more familiar

English versions are preferred to Nomina Anatomica)

C *sistem saraf simpati* (my sympathy to proponents of this term)

D *sistem saraf bersimpati* (bigger sympathy for this one)

So how was that? Too easy? Hmm . . . are you guys truly bilingual now, or what? Trilingual you say (including Latin!) . . . some say more, with Hokkien, Tamil, Esperanto, Doctorspeak (Technobabble) etc, etc. What can I say . . . but that I'm overjoyed, now that our mission to see through the PM's vision to promote multilingualism is nearing 20/20! At the same time however, we have to forge ahead in elevating the status of Bahasa Malaysia from a mere unifier of the races to a **competent** language of science and technology and the professions. It may well become the *lingua franca* of Asean—*Bahasa* Asean.

God bless Malaysia . . . *MERDEKA!*

*   *   *

UPDATE 10
HUKUM D-M

Just as the mass media is abuzz these days with *Hukum Hudud, Berita MMA* (the "mess" media for doctors since 1991 AU . . . After Update) wants to splash up this month of September with *Hukum D-M*. Just as *Hukum Hudud* comes with its attendant speculation on hand surgery, and association with the Opposition, *Hukum D-M* triggers the suspicion that it might be the Prime Minister's latest brainchild: *Hukum Dr Mahathir* (Dr M's Law). I hate to disappoint you guys but *Hukum D-M* (D-M Rule) has got nothing to do with Dr M or the Malaysian Government. It has everything to do with one Prof Sutan Takdir Alisjahbana who introduced this concept in his book *Tatabahasa Baru Bahasa Melayu / Indonesia* (New Grammar in the Malay / Indonesian Language) . . . which practically says: "Tata" Bahasa or ("Bye-bye" Bahasa)! Hmmmm

So what the heck is Hukum D-M?

Hukum D-M was introduced to sort out the confusion surrounding the translation of complex terms with multiple adjectives from English to *Bahasa Malaysia*. In *Hukum D-M*, the **D** represents **'Diterang'** (the **describee**, usually a noun) and the **M** stands for **'Menerang'** (the **describer** ie the adjective that qualifies the noun). So, by *Hukum D-M* we can see that the describee (or the described) comes before the describer, ie noun before adjective for example: **Klinik Mata (Eye Clinic).** Now that's easy enough because the term consists of only two words. The fun begins when we have a string of adjectives like a few of those in the Kuizria last month, which needless to say must have baffled the gray matter out of some of you. Yes . . . this *Hukum D-M* is the promised input on the rules of translating terms comprising two or more words. As always (OK . . . 99.99% of the time), I am true to my words.

Let's recap what you did with the 20 questions:

Q 10 blood (M) vessel (D) = pembuluh (D) darah (M)

Q 12 acute (M) arthritis (D) = artritis (D) akut (M)

Q 13 automatic (M) bar (D) = palang (D) automatic (M)

Q 14 local (M) anesthesia (D) = anestesia (D) setempat (M)

Q 15 clinical (M) examination (D) = pemeriksaan (D) klinikal (M)

Q 17 collapsing (M) pulse (D) = nadi (D) melenyap (M)

The above terms comprise only two words and are therefore very straightforward. You simply cannot go wrong here. Just reverse the English M-D (Adjective-Noun) to the equivalent *Bahasa D-M* (Noun-Adjective).

Q 18 common cold = *selesema*

This is another instance where you just can't go wrong syntax-wise (but you can still mess up the spelling!)

because there's nothing to sequence as the *Bahasa* equivalent is only one word.

Q 4 autoantibody = *autoantibodi*

I said that 'bodi anti auto' would be correct if 'autoantibody' were three separate words. There is a tendency these days to split what is a one-word terminology in English into its components for instance a few people would just love to dissect **endoscopy** (Q 7) into 'endo (M) + scopy (D)', giving the ridiculous *Bahasa* equivalent of *'skop (D) dalaman (M)'*; or worse, *skop (D) endo (M)*, and this would be a poor attempt at the definition rather than the term (**'endoskopi'**). In view of the aforesaid malpractice, I have emphasized that technical terms need only be given spellchange treatment **for example: *mikroskop*** (for **microscope**) not *'skop mikro'*. (Of course there's always the usual exceptions such as ***gelombang mikro*** for **microwave**. I would prefer 'mikrowav', but who am I . . . but a humble Updater . . . to prefer this or that?).

Q 11 midstream urine (MSU) = *(air) kencing aliran tengah*

We have a situation here that is somewhat similar to 'common cold' above, where the number of words per terminology in the two languages are not the same. While in 'common cold' we have one word less in Bahasa, here in MSU it's the opposite. But the D-M Rule still holds where D is *(air) kencing* (for **urine**) and M is *aliran tengah* (for **midstream**). It is unfortunate that Bahasa still lacks a number of the abbreviated forms such as 'mid' which can nicely be joined to another word to coin a brand new term using just one word. So why not 'midstrim' as in option A? Well . . . this is again a matter of **who** is coining the word in question. That is why it is quite alright for Linguists & Co. to bury words like *penyunting* (in favor of/IFO *editor*), *ungkapan* (IFO *frasa*), *takrifan* (IFO *definisi*), *mutu* (IFO *kualiti*), *bahas* (IFO *debat*), *maktab* (IFO *kolej*), *sejadi* (IFO *natural*, pronounced 'nah-too-rahl') . . . I can go on forever . . . *piawai* (IFO *standard*, pronounced 'stun-dud'! I know you're stunned dead because I can hear a thud!!) Yet Medicine is strongly 'persuaded' to use *kambuh* instead of (i/o) *relaps, bentan* i/o *rekrudesens, pelopor* i/o *prakursor, tumbung* i/o *prolaps, daun telinga* i/o *aurikel, salah amat* i/o *ilusi, goiter ringkas* i/o *goiter simpel, kemaluan* i/o *pudendum* . . . (a headmaster once declared **in shame** during the school assembly, upon the misbehavior of one of his students: *"Amat besarlah **kemaluan** saya atas apa yang telah berlaku"* . . .). Only time can tell which terms will survive and thrive. So it's up to you users.

Q 20. sympathetic nervous system
= *sistem saraf simpatetik*

Generally, the more familiar English versions are preferred to Nomina Anatomica which in this case would be **systema nervorum sympathicum**. However, you'll notice that *sistema nervorum simpatikum*, the *Bahasa* equivalent of the Latin version, follows the same sequence as *sistem saraf simpatetik*. In other words, Latin syntax is the same as that of *Bahasa Malaysia*. This means that we don't have to worry about the sequencing when we translate popular Latin terms such as **status asthmaticus (*status asmatikus*—Q 16), hyperemesis gravidarum *(hiperemesis gravidarum)*, anorexia nervosa *(anoreksia nervosa)*, paralysis agitans *(paralisis agitans)*, delirium tremens *(delirium*** *tremens)*, **larva migrans** *(larva migrans)*, **abductor pollicis longus** *(abduktor polisis longus)*, and so on. However, what you had in Q 19 **grand mal epilepsy** is a mixture of Latin ('grand mal') and English ('epilepsy'). So we have to take it one step at a time to analyze the components. The M here is 'grand mal' and the D is 'epilepsy'. So all we have to do is reverse it to D-M and that's how we got **epilepsi grand mal.** 'Wrong sequence' was the comment given to option C *epilepsi mal grand*, because the Latin component 'grand mal' was reversed as though it was English.

Common Errors

Because we are not familiar with *Hukum D-M*, mistakes occur when it comes to translating 3-word (or more) terminologies. Notorious ones include *kadar kasar kematian* **(crude death rate)** when it should be **kadar kematian kasar**, just as **gross national product** is **keluaran negara kasar,** not *keluaran kasar negara*. Several **general post offices** in the country had been advertising their mistakes *(pejabat besar pos)* in huge signboards for years until recently when they were rectified to **pejabat pos besar.** I'm sure at this point many of you are foaming at the mouth with counter arguments such as "How can the *kematian* be *kasar?*

It's the *kadar* that is *kasar!*" Point taken. But it's funny how we have no trouble at all with **'fresh cows' milk'.** We do not fuss that "It's the milk that's fresh, not the cows". And rightly so too 'cos cows don't get fresh. They can't . . . even if they want to . . . this is the prerogative of the bulls!

Teori Unsur Terdekat (TUT)

To cut the bull (tut-tut!) so serious academic discussion can resume on a professional level, let us examine a few examples: Let's look as **'blood films'** *(filem darah)* . . . make that '**thin** blood films' *(filem darah tipis)*. See how logical it becomes when you build the term up in stages. We can actually analyse this using Hukum D-M. In 'thin blood film' we know the main component (D) is 'film' *(filem)* ie the noun. Then we qualify it (with the M component) by saying it's a **blood** film, not X-ray film *(filem darah bukan filem X-ray)*. We may ask further, "what type of blood film?" Answer: "**Thin** blood film, not thick *(filem darah **tipis**, bukan tebal)*". At this stage, 'thin' is the M qualifying 'blood film' (the D). It's as if there is a hierachy of qualifiers (or adjectives). Coming back to the argument of whether *kasar* qualifies *kadar* or *kematian*, the answer is neither: using the D-M rule, *kematian (M)* qualifies *kadar (D)* giving us *kadar kematian.* Take it one step further and ask the question "What type of *kadar kematian?*" . . . the answer is *kadar kematian 'yang kasar'* or just *kadar kematian kasar* ie *'kasar' (M)* qualifies *'kadar kematian' (D)*, not *kadar* alone. It's like as if *'kasar'* is the second echelon qualifier, and should therefore be one position further in rank than the first echelon qualifier *'kematian'* in relation to the main component *'kadar'*. This is ***'Teori Unsur Terdekat'*** **(Closest Component Theory)** (which takes the D-M concept one step further) and is better visualized schematically as shown below for **Malaysian crude death rate:**

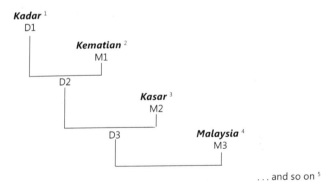

Fig 1: *Teori Unsur Terdekat*

I hope it's crystal clear now that the describee (D) / noun comes before the describer / qualifier (M) as spelt out by *Hukum D-M*, and that the primary qualifier (M1) is closest to the noun (D), followed by the other qualifiers in ranking order (M2, M3, M4 and so on) in line with the **Teori Unsur Terdekat.**

Exceptions

Now that the D-M haze is cleared up, we can look at the omnipresent exceptions which is the rule with most linguistics rules . . . after all these are not the Ten Commandments. Exceptions are sequenced as M-D instead of D-M. Classics include the hot favorite of tourists, the **goreng pisang** (M-D) when it should strictly be **pisang goreng** (D-M) which somehow doesn't sound too hot. How about **kesan dadah mudarat (adverse drug reactions?)** *Kesan dadah mudarat* is rather woolly as it may mean either **kesan mudarat** of **dadah** or **kesan** of **dadah mudarat**. This is one example where you'd have to doctor the original English to the 'X of Y' form to avoid ambiguities. In this case, we can transform the original English version to **'adverse reactions of drugs'** rather than 'adverse drug reactions'. Translated, 'adverse reactions of drugs' becomes **kesan mudarat dadah** (not *kesan mudarat <u>dari</u> dadah* though, as the conjunction 'of' does not require any translation in *Bahasa Malaysia*).

Another one is **Perdana Menteri** *(M-D)*. I suppose in preMerdeka days, not many people knew of *Hukum D-M* (. . . . so what's changed?) And with the heavy influence of the British with their *Hukum M-D,* (which persists until today in **Cekap Express, 2-minit mi, Minah Restoran, Veedayan Kedai Video, Loh Bak Kong Kedai Keranda,** etc, etc), we elected to have a *Perdana Menteri* rather than a *Menteri Perdana.*

I wonder how the **Prime Minister** feels about being called the *Menteri Perdana* of Malaysia. On second thought, we'll let him stay as *Perdana Menteri* or we'll get a dose of *Hukum Dr M!* Until next month, **"Selamat menyambut hari keputeraan Nabi"** and happy updating.

*   *   *

REFERENCES

1   *Senarai Istilah Umum Perubatan dan Kesihatan. Bahasa Inggeris—Bahasa Malaysia.* Dewan Bahasa dan Pustaka, Cetakan Pertama, 1982

2   *Senarai Istilah Farmasi dan Farmakologi. Bahasa Inggeris—Bahasa Malaysia.* Dewan Bahasa dan Pustaka, Cetakan Pertama, 1982

3   *Senarai Ejaan Rumi Bahasa Malaysia,* Dewan Bahasa dan Pustaka, Cetakan Kelapan, 1988

4   *Kamus Dewan Edisi Baru.* Dewan Bahasa dan Pustaka, Cetakan Pertama, 1989

5   *Istilah Perubatan Bahasa Inggeris—Bahasa Malaysia.* Dewan Bahasa dan Pustaka, Cetakan Ketiga, 1990.

6   *Kamus Perubatan* disunting oleh Nik Aziz Sulaiman, Nor Azila Adnan, Edariah Abu Bakar, Siti Aishah Md Ali, Noresah Baharom dan Hasnah Mohamed. Dewan Bahasa dan Pustaka, Cetakan Pertama 1991